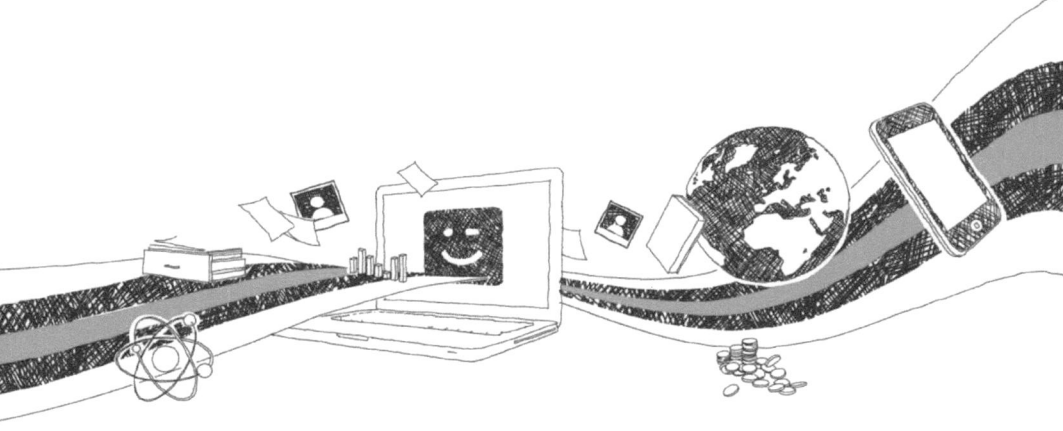
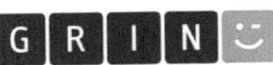

Bibliographic information published by the German National Library:

The German National Library lists this publication in the National Bibliography;
detailed bibliographic data are available on the Internet at http://dnb.dnb.de .

Imprint:

Copyright © 2019 GRIN Verlag
Print and binding: Books on Demand GmbH, Norderstedt Germany
ISBN: 9783346080875

This book at GRIN:

https://www.grin.com/document/510518

Adane Shalamo

Solid Waste Management in Emerging Towns of Ethiopia. A Research Proposal

GRIN Verlag

GRIN - Your knowledge has value

Since its foundation in 1998, GRIN has specialized in publishing academic texts by students, college teachers and other academics as e-book and printed book. The website www.grin.com is an ideal platform for presenting term papers, final papers, scientific essays, dissertations and specialist books.

Visit us on the internet:

http://www.grin.com/

http://www.facebook.com/grincom

http://www.twitter.com/grin_com

HAWSSA UNIVERSITY

COLLEGE OF MEDICINE AND HEALTH SCIENCES SCHOOL OF PUBLIC AND
ENVIRONMENTAL HEALTH DEPARTMENT OF ENVIRONMENTAL HEALTH

ASSESSMENT OF STEERET SOLID WASTE MANAGEMENT PRACTICES AND
ASSOCIATED FACTORS IN HAWASSA CITY, SOUTHERN, ETHIOPIA 2019

A RESEARCH PROPOSAL SUBMITTED TO THE SCHOOL OF PUBLIC AND
ENVIRONMENTAL HEALTH IN PARTIAL FULFILLMENT OF THE REQUIREMENTS
FOR THE DEGREE OF MASTER OF PUBLIC HEALTH IN ENVIRONMENTAL HEALTH

HAWASSA, ETHIOPIA

HAWSSA UNIVERSITY

FACULITY OF HEALTH SCIENCES

SCHOOL OF PUBLIC AND ENVIRONMENTAL HEALTH

Table of Contents

ACKNOWLEDGEMENT

First of all, I would like to thank the almighty of God who brought me to being and help to pass through up and down of life until today.

I would like to express my appreciation to my advisor Dr. Hunachew Beyene who equipped me with scientific research writing skill that helps me in making this proposal as such productive and Mr. Dawit Derese for their unreserved encouragement, provision relevant comments and guidance give on my works.

Also I would like to acknowledge the Hawassa University, collage of medicine and health science school of environmental health give me a chance will be conducted this study.

List of Table

List of Figures

List of Abbreviations and Acronym

CI	confidence interval
DE	Design Effect
ETB	Ethiopian Birr
FDRE	Federal democratic republic of Ethiopia
FGD	Focus group discussion
HH	Household
MSSE	micro and small scale enterprises
MSW	Municipal solid waste
MSWM	Municipal solid waste management
RS	Random sampling
SBPDD	sanitation, beautification and parks development department
S.N	Serial number
SEPH	Socio-economic profile of Hawassa city
SPSS	Statistical package for social science
SW	Solid Waste
SWM	Solid Waste Management
SNNPR	southern nation nationality peoples region
NGO'S	Non-Governmental organizations
WTP	willing to pay

Summary

Background: Street Solid waste causes substantial harm to the environment and human health if mismanaged. Which is a consequence of day-to-day activity of human kind, needs to be managed properly. With rapid urbanization and population growth problems related to Street solid waste management have become considerable importance in Ethiopia from both environment and human safety. This urges for a better understanding of the current practices and problems of street solid waste management in emerging towns of Ethiopia.

Objectives:

The objective of this study will be to assess the current street solid waste management practices and its associated factors in Hawassa city, southern Ethiopia.

Methods and materials: A community-based Cross- sectional study will be conducted in the city of Hawassa from February 2 to March 13th by using stratified sampling, systematic random sampling, and purposive sampling techniques. From three Kebeles, further information from responsible staff using interviews, FGD and field observation. A total 543 study subjects will be recruited and their street waste management practices and associated factors will be evaluated. Data will be collected through both quantitative and qualitative methods. Six data a collectors with a public health background will be used to collect data. Data will be entered and cleaned using Epi info version 7 and export to SPSS version 21 computer software for further analysis. Determinants of street solid waste managements will be explained by Descriptive statistics (frequencies, proportions) to describe the study subjects. The logistic regression technique will be used. The result will be presented in statements, tables, and charts. Finally in all analysis, p-value < 0.05 will be considered as significant.

Budge break down: Total budget needed for study will account 30673.10 ETB.

Key words –Street Solid waste, its associated factors and Solid waste Management, Hawassa

1. Introduction

1.1. Background

The human activities which take place in this world create waste. The wastes could be both solid and liquid types and the way they are going to be handled, stored and disposed of can expose the environment and public health to risks. Solid waste management includes all activities that seek to minimize health, environmental and aesthetic impacts of solid waste in urban areas. In urban areas, Solid waste generated by domestic households, commercial and industrial enterprise, health care and institutional activities, as well as on the streets. The Street waste contains a mixture of waste from many sources, because streets are used dumping ground by all generators of wastes where sanitation facilities are lacking and a large animal population roams the streets, it also contains a lot of human fecal matter, manure and often used for extensive dumping of construction and demolition debris attracting further dumping of solid waste (1).

Solid waste management is one of the most important environmental services and integrated part of basic urban services. Study conducted in Kenya showed that approximately 50 per cent of solid waste generated daily in Nairobi is disposed of unsafely. Poor solid waste management (SWM) has negative health impacts, including the proliferation of infectious and non-communicable diseases. It also contributes to environmental degradation and greenhouse gas emissions (2). The situation implies that Solid Waste Management task is becoming series concern due to the alarming rate of population growth and development of urbanization in the world (3).

The problem associated with Solid Waste Management in today's societies is complex because of the quantitative and diverse nature of waste. The development of extensive urban areas and the finding limitation for public service in many cities the impact of technologies and raw materials(4). Solid Waste Management is a problem that experienced by all countries in the world it is the issue mostly witnessed in urban areas as a result of a high surge in population growth rate and increase in per capital income. This poising danger to environmental quality and human health (5).because of its nature, it has remained one of the major environmental problems of human beings continue to face.

High population rate and increase income activities in urban area of developing countries combined with lack of train in modern Solid Waste Management practices complicated the efforts to improve the Solid Waste Management services in developing countries the per-capital generation of Solid Waste Management in urban areas is much less compared with the developed countries; however, the capacity of developing countries to collect, process, dispose and reuse the Solid Waste in a cost-effective manner is significantly limited compared with the developed countries(6).

SWM is one of the basic services that are currently receiving wide attention in many towns in Ethiopia. This is mainly because; SWM that is generated in the most town of Ethiopia is not appropriately handled and managed(7). The Municipality and other stake holders in Ethiopia have overall responsibility for Solid Waste Management in their town and cities. However, most of them are failed to fulfill their responsibilities especially sound way of dealing with the waste genera ration, collection, transport, treatment and disposal (8).

Moreover, according to a preliminary survey conducted by the researcher solid wastes in Hawassa city are observed on the road, open areas, street, ditches, and river and disposed in sewerage. But the solid waste management, particularly at street level, is not managed in a well-organized manner. This implies that, like other developing country cities, Hawassa` have also problems that prevent the municipality responsible body from doing its task for environmental sound with economic efficiency. So, this research is intended to identify and analyze the main determinants of solid waste management practice at street level.

1.2. Statement of the Problem

Urbanization with inadequate waste management practices, specifically, widespread disposal of waste in water bodies, dumping inside the road and uncontrolled dump sites aggravates the problems of generally low sanitation levels across the African countries including Ethiopia(9).

Hawassa city is characterized by rapid population growth caused by natural increase and rural urban migration. Such rapid increase in population together with rapid development of the town has produced increasing volumes of solid waste and in turn it induced greater infrastructural demand, institutional setup and community participation for its management. But, the town sanitation, beautification and parks development department (SBPDD) which runs the solid waste management activities of the town could not fulfill the above requirements. For instance, currently SBPDD has practice its activity by supplying one skip loader, tractors, three-wheel cars for collection, transportation and disposal of the town solid waste. In addition to this, there are no public solid waste storage containers and road side dust bins. So that it highly suffered from shortage of solid waste management infrastructures and faced unmatched burdens of collection, transportation and disposal of solid wastes. Furthermore, SBPDD is surrounded by different institutional constraints such as lack of sufficient waste collection vehicles, weak financial and material resource, weak regulation and controlling mechanism, and insignificant movement for public awareness creation.

These limitations led to deterioration of the town environment and also reinforce incorrect disposal habits to the people. Most of solid wastes that are generated in the town remain uncollected and simply dumped in open areas, road sides, river courses, ditches. According to the report made by municipality of Hawassa city in 2018, the total solid waste generated in 2018 is estimated to be 190-250 ton/day(10).

From this amount more than 150-200 ton/day (80%) of solid wastes were collected and transported but the rest (20%) was discarded into streets, drains, ditches, canals and open spaces; slums and squatter settlers of the town population mostly lacks any form of solid waste collection services, and disposed of their solid wastes into roadsides(10).

The Final disposal method is also open dumping type which widely practiced in many developing countries and has hazardous effect on health and the environment. Besides this, current disposal site is a closed quarry site in the city and open dumping and lack of establishment of waste management system based on actually waste generation amount and quantitative data.

As a result, municipal solid waste management in Hawassa has not been carried out in a sufficient and proper manner. The environmental and sanitary conditions of the town have become more serious from time to time, and people are suffering from living in such conditions. So that urgent need of efficient MSWM on one hand and steady growth of solid waste problem on the other side are still the main features of the city.

Most studies conducted so far in line with this study give more emphasis the issues directly or indirectly on provision of services to manage MSW. However, there is little study that considers street solid waste management practices. Therefore, this study aims to assessing street solid waste management and associated factors of the study area.

1.3. Literature review

As study conducted in Nigeria indicate that poor waste management practices among residents include open dumping, practiced by 66.3% of the residents and burning as practiced by 62.4% of respondents(11).

Result revealed that 61.0% of the HHs disposed of their waste at community bins or had waste picked up at their homes by private contractors. The remaining 39.0% disposed of their waste in gutters, streets, holes and nearby bushes as study conducted in Accra (12).

As study conducted in Somalia The findings revealed that Karan district community have good level of knowledge as well as have positive attitude but their practice towards solid waste management was poor (13).

The study done in Bahir Dar indicate that (40%) of disposed wastes illegally at the road sides and open fields, 19.4% of households burned their collected wastes, 8.9% buried them inside their compounds, 5.1% disposed them in and around these compounds, 8.9% simply disposed the waste in the compounds, and the remaining 17.7% dumped them at river side's (14).

The study conducted in Bahirdar the results showed that 66.6% practice illegal solid waste disposal with the remaining 33.4% waiting until solid waste collectors come to the area to take the waste away (14).

The study conducted in Dire Dawa town the result of multivariate analysis showed that (69%) disposed solid wastes in improper manner (15).

As Study conducted in Asella town result revealed that (82.8%), had improper solid waste management practice(16).

1.3.4. Factors associated with Solid waste management practices

1.3.4.1 Demographic factors

In sirilqanka the logistic regression results revealed that household size and household expenditure significantly and positively influences the household willingness to pay. Quantity of waste generated, number of times disposing the waste and gender had a negative coefficient and were significant $(p<0.05)(17)$.

As study conducted in Thailand revealed that a significant association was found between sex and solid waste management behavior. This indicated that male were almost two times more likely to have poor solid waste management behavior (18).

A Study done in Thailand result showed that the association between education level and solid waste management behavior was significant. This indicated that the respondents who had been educated in secondary and above were almost two times more likely to have poor solid waste management behavior (18).

As study conducted in Thailand the results showed that the odds of currently being solid waste manage of family size above five is less than one implying that about 75.9 (18).

The study conducted in Nigeria showed that Gender and educational status of respondents significantly influenced their knowledge, attitude and practice of waste management p < 0.05 (11).

In Bahirdar results of multiple linear regressions showed that household size and household total income were determinate factors of household's solid waste generation (14).

According to research done in Debrebirhan the result showed that odds of currently being solid waste manage for primary education level are 2 time the odds uneducated level of currently being solid waste manage(19).

According to finding in debrebirhan The coefficient of year of stay is negative indicating that when the year of stay is decrease by one year then to dispose solid waste manage is decrease by 4%(19).

In Dire Dawa results showed that about 31% are disposing solid waste in a proper manner. This implies that respondents who are illiterate were 2times more likely to be improper when compared to those who are literate (20).

The study conducted in Diredawa town result showed that Households their average monthly income less than or equal to 3,000ETB were 0.5times less likely to be improper compared to those greater than 3,000ETB.This showed that when the average monthly incomes of the household increase and the tendency to be improperly manage solid waste was also increase(20)

Some literatures showed that the higher income leads peoples to more participation domestic solid waste management because, the higher income earner groups have a power to use the service of private waste collectors at any cost than the lower income group(11).

A study conducted in dire dawa the results showed that Household who family size greater than five people were 0.4times less likely to be improper when compared to those who is less than or equal to four people. This indicates that households who manage solid wastes properly have, relatively, a large number of family members than households who manage its waste improperly (20).

As study conducted in diredawa finding indicated that respondents who live < 1year in current HH were 0.5times less likely to be improper when compared to those who live greater or equal to 1 year (20).

The study conducted diredawa the results shows that Respondents who are not married were 1.6 times more likely to be improper when compared to those who are. This implies the majority (72.7%) of the respondents were married (20).

The study conducted in shashemene revealed that while the ages of the respondents increase by 1%, willingness to pay is reduced by 0.59%. This implies that younger respondents would know and appreciate the value of SWM than the older ones about the negative impacts of solid wastes, Household size has also negatively significant ($p<0.5$) effect on Willing To Pay Similarly, marginal effect indicates that all factors keeping constant, at 1% increase of the household size of the respondents; their willingness to pay is reduced by 7.47%Income has a positive relationship with the households WTP ($p<0.05$). This indicates that improved SWM is a normal good since its demand increases with income. This implies households with high income are more willing to Pay for the SWM than households with low incomes. This indicates while household income increases by 1 Ethiopian birr, WTP for SWM improvement increases by 0.01%,Education has positive coefficients and significance at $p < 0.05$.An increase in the respondents year of schooling by 1% will increase their willingness to pay for improved SWM services by 18.31%(21).

1.3.4.2.Socio-cultural factors

As study conducted in Thailand the result showed that significant association between knowledge and solid waste management behavior. This indicated that respondents who had a low level of solid waste management knowledge were almost three times more likely to commit poor solid waste management behavior. It also finding showed that there was an association between attitudes of solid waste management and good solid waste management behavior. This indicated that the respondent who had poor attitude levels toward solid waste management were three times more likely to have poor behavior in solid waste management. Attitude toward solid waste management was the strongest factor to predict separation behavior and recycling behavior (18).

A study done in Malaysia indicated that knowledge is an important factor to predict solid waste separation behavior and it also finding revealed that attitude toward waste management is the strongest factor that is related to waste management behaviors (22).

Finding showed that 94.2% were aware of hazards brought about by incorrect solid waste management yet only 26.2% practiced correct management methods as study done in Kenya (22).

A study conduct in Nigeria the results showed that 90% of respondents were aware of waste management while 97.5% had positive attitude towards it (23).

A study conducted at Nigeria the results indicated that large generation at high rate without a corresponding efficient technology to manage the wastes,35.8% respondents used waste collection services, 64.2% used other waste disposal options, 16.4% used both, 68.7% and 58.7% were aware of waste collection service and waste management regulations, respectively; while 28.4% separated their solid wastes at source(24).

Injibara town, The finding indicated that 81.06% were willing to pay for the service (25).

results showed that The odds of currently no awareness about solid waste manage technique is less than one implying about 81.2% as compared with communities who have awareness about solid waste manage as study done in debrebrhan (19).

A Study conducted dire dawa result showed that Respondents who are not aware about solid waste management were 3.8times more likely to be improper compared to those who have knowledge. This Indicated that the level of household's awareness on extensive implication of improper waste management increases, the probability of effective solid waste management at household level would be increased by 17%. (20).

The studies conducted in diredawa result showed that respondent who have poor attitude towards solid waste management were 1.7times more likely to be improper when compared to those who are good attitude (20).

As Study conducted in mizanamane result showed that 81.8% of the respondents have good knowledge, 77.5% of the participants showed positive attitude toward waste management as well as 76.9% of participants have good practice to ward waste management (26).

1.3.4.3. Institutional factors

The study conducted in Thailand results revealed that respondent who had not received information about solid waste management were almost two times more likely to have poor solid waste management behavior; this indicated that the respondents who are better informed about solid waste management information likely have better solid waste management behavior (27).

A study conducted in Bahir Dar showed that results indicating that 78% of the respondents feel that the current solid waste management service is far below the required level; whereas, 22% of the respondents show satisfaction with the existing waste management service also, results indicating that solid waste management service for the residents once a week, but the survey results demonstrate that only 29% of the sample households received solid waste management services weekly, indicating that the performance of solid waste management service is low(14).

A study conducted in Debrebirhan results showed that the odds ratios of currently being solid waste manage for implementation of government policy is less than one about 83.6% as compared with doesn't implementation government policy(19) .

The study conducted in diredawa results showed that the Law enforcement respondents when the regulation weak were 2.8 times more likely to be improperly manage waste than when the regulation becomes strong which indicated positive relationship between effective solid waste management and enforcement of regulation (20).

A study conducted in dire dawa results showed that the households who have no access to MSSE were five times more likely to be improper when compared to those accesses of MSSE. Similar studies revealed that households who have no access to MSSE were 18times more likely to be improper when compared to those access of MSSE service and also accesses to private waste collectors showed significant relation with household waste management (20).

As Study conducted in Asella town result revealed that Participants who didn't have access to door to door solid waste collection service were about three times more likely to practice improper solid waste management when compared to those who had access (AOR = 2.873, 95 CI (1.565,5.273) P = 0.001(16).

Technical Factors

A study carried out in Nairobi and Mombasa revealed that high variability in SWM practices, from storage to collection, transport and disposal. Residents of both cities who participated in the study reported high levels of awareness about health risks associated with poor SWM, yet limited awareness of waste reduction, reuse and recycling (2).

A study conducted in debrebirhan results showed that the odd of currently being solid waste manage for the not willing to pay for waste collectors is less than about 60.9%odds of currently being solid waste manage to not enough access for waste storage are greater than one about 9 times the odds of currently being solid waste manage for no evidence about the waste storage around their village Enough access is greater than one about three as compared to the reference of none (19).

A study conducted in Bahir Dar results showed that the only (47.3%) households received solid waste management services by municipality waste collectors weekly. While (16%) households, (25.9%) households,(10.7%) households received solid waste management services within 15 days, 21 days and once in a month, respectively, and (43%) residents never received solid waste collection, transportation and final disposal in to landfill services the Only 31% of sample households have separate bins and the remaining households do not have separate bins for storage of different types of waste separately for simple waste management purpose (14).

The study conducted in Jimma town results indicated that "lack of infrastructure for collection, transportation, treatment and disposal of solid waste, proper solid waste management planning, insufficient financial resources, technical expertise and public attitude has made the situation aggravating due to several environmental and health-related problems are increasing.(28)

A study conducted in wolayta sodo results revealed that the current SWM practices and services at both HH and municipality level of Wolaita Sodo town was weak in terms of status as well as spatial coverage and service delivery is entangled by many very serious problems(29).

A study conducted in hosanna town the result indicated that widespread practice of open dumping due to lack of appropriate facilities for solid waste management (30).

1.5. Conceptual frame work

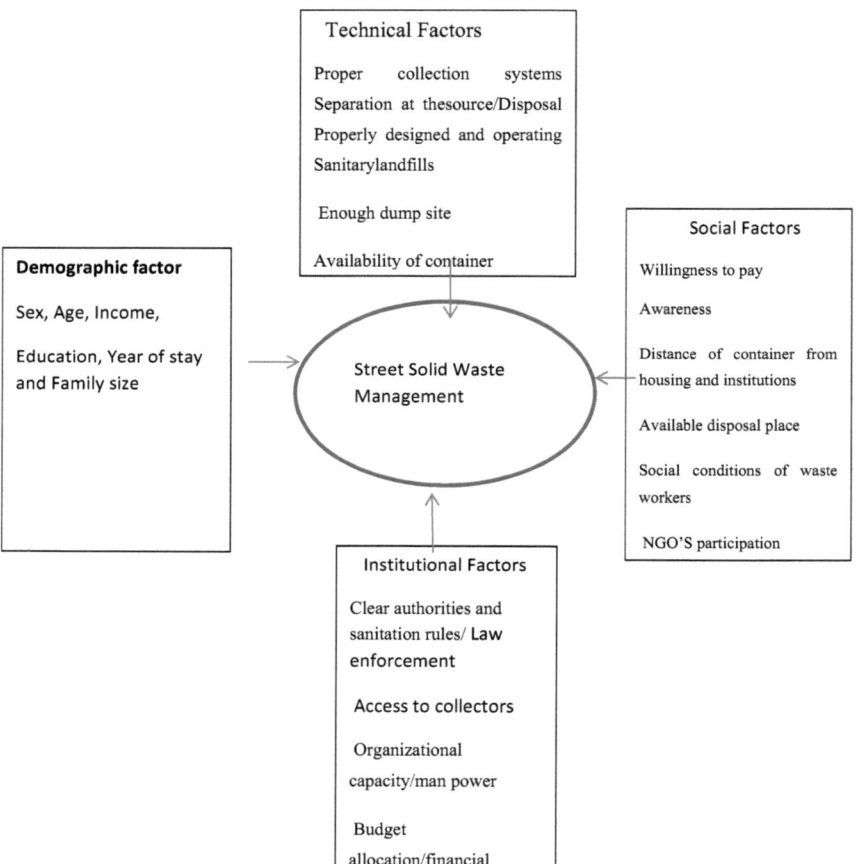

Figure 1- frame work showing all possible factors indicated in literature review adopted from different literatures, Hawassa city,2019.

1.6. Basic research questions:

By having the above mentioned reasons to do, the following basic research questions will be answered by the researcher in the study.

1. What does the current street solid waste management practice of the town look like?

2. What are the factors affecting street solid waste management practices in the city

1.7. Significance of the study

The result of this research will help inspectors and stakeholders in solid waste management and disposal practices. In addition, to indicate how to involve the community and institutions in the solid waste management and disposal practices.

Furthermore, it can help Hawassa city municipality to have strong action plan and policies on street SWM practices.

It will also help policy makers, researchers and environmental protection agencies as guideline information to improve current existing solid waste management problems and to minimize related problems.

In addition to this, it will provides baseline information for non-governmental organization and decision makers to prepare action plan for further implementation and to develop proper solid waste management practices strategy at all levels.

2. Objectives

2.1. General objective

- To assess the current practices and associated factors of street solid waste management in Hawassa city, southern Ethiopia, 2019/20.

2.2. Specific Objectives

➢ To assess the current practices of street solid waste management in Hawassa city, southern Ethiopia, 2019/20.

➢ To identify the factors that affects the street solid waste management practice in Hawassa city southern Ethiopia, 2019/20.

3. Methodology

3.1. Study Area

Hawassa is located in the southern nation's nationalities and peoples region on the shores of Lake Hawassa in the Great Rift Valley, 273km south of Addis Ababa and 1125kms north of Nairobi, Kenya. The city lays between 6° 55' 0'' to 7° 6' 0'' latitude north and 38° 25' 0'' to 38° 34' 0'' longitudes east. Hawassa city is bounded by Lake Hawassa in the west, oromia region in the north, wondogenet woreda in the east and shebedino woreda in the south. Hawassa is serving as the capital of southern nation's nationalities and peoples region, the sidama zone administration and Hawassa city administration.

The city administration has an area of 157.2sq.kms and it has eight sub cities and thirty two kebeles. These eight sub-cities are Hayke dare, Meneharia, Tabor, Misrak, BahileAderash, Addis Ketema, Hawela-Tula and Mehal sub- city (31).

3.1.2 Demographic characteristics

According to 2007 national census report, the town had 258,808 total populations while in the estimated population in 2015 it reached 357,000 and 2017 was about 390,000 peoples a with growth rate of 3.5%/annually. Based on 2018, estimated total population 390,000 out of this

194220 male and 195780 are female. While 242489 are living in the urban area, the rest of population living rural area. A total of 61,279 households were counted in the town(10).

The socio- economic development of the town is very encouraging; the town contains 147 schools out of this 51 kindergarten 41 primary schools and 36 junior school 5-8 grades, secondary school 9-10, 13 Preparatory school 11-12 grades, in which 2 is governmental school and the rest 11 are non-governmental school, and . In addition to that the town has 3 government and 6 non-governmental hospitals and 15 public health keeping center, 51 private clinics, and 55 pharmacies and 46 drug stores with 2 diagnostic laboratories(31).

Hawassa is one of the most attractive towns in Ethiopia, Exploring the town is an enjoyable and worthwhile experience for both foreign and domestic tourists. Among the tourist attractions in the town the major one is Lake Hawassa, Gudumale, AmoraGedel, MtTabor, Mt Alamura, and spring water.

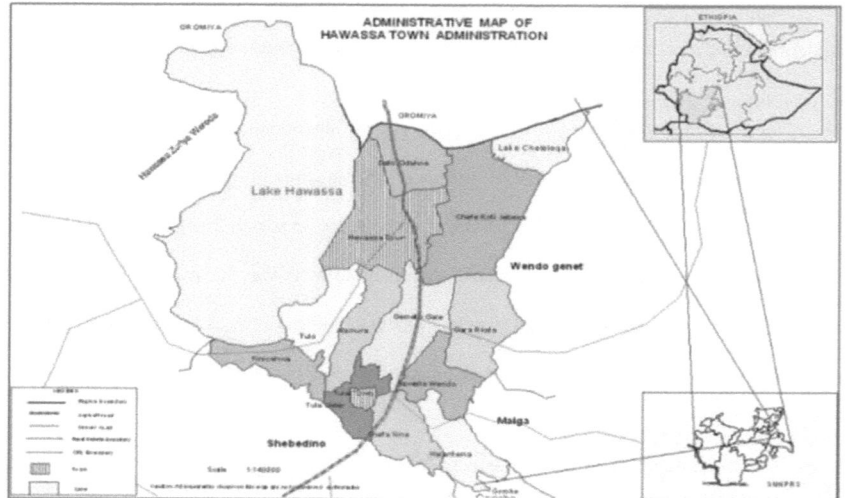

Figure 2 - Hawassa city administrative division map

Source : Hawassa city administration finance office, 2019

3.2. Study Design and period

Mixed research design approach, which will followed descriptive survey method approach incorporating qualitative and quantitative research design. will be used from November 14 to May 24, 2019 in Hawassa city.

3. 3.Study Population

3.3.1. A source population will be all households which registered by Kebeles administrative units in Hawassa city.

3.3.2. The study population will be those household heads or household members represented from selected HH with in their respective Kebeles during the study period.

3.3.3. Study sample
All randomly selected HHs in selected Keble will be included in the study.

3.3.4. The study unit
The study unit will be the head of the house.

3.4. Inclusion and exclusion of population

3.4.1. Inclusion criteria
All sampled households and those aged above 18 years, house wives, house band or other family of household will be included in the study.

3.4.2. Exclusion criteria
Households who cannot respond the questionnaire due to illness, social and individual problems will be excluded. /household heads lived for less than 6 months in the selected Kebeles will exclude for the study.

3.5. Sample Size and Sampling Procedures

3.5.1. Sample Size

Current status of street solid waste management practice in Hawassa city will be calculated by using scientific statistical method from (32).

The sample size (n) for the first objective is calculated using single population formula based on assumption of 31% proportion (P) which was done on Dire Dawa city.

P =31% proportion of HHs expected to practice proper household solid waste management (20).

A standard z score of 1.96 corresponding to Confidence interval of 95%; Margin of error (d) = 0.05; Non-response rate = 10%; DE of 1.5 to provide correction which will result from sampling error.

Accordingly, the sample size calculated will be:

$n=Z (\alpha/2)^2 P (1-P)/d^2$ $n= (1.96)^2 x0.31 (1-0.31)/ (0.05)^2 =3.84*0.8217/0.0025= 328.6$

Accordingly the required sample size $=(328.6*1.5) + 10\% = 542.19 =543$

By adding 10% of non-response and multiplying the sample size by 1.5 for DE of the sample size will be increased to 543 respondents (households).

Second objective sample size will determined based on identified factors by a study conducted in Dire Dawa City, Debre Birhan, Addis Ababa

The sample size for first objectives will measured to be 328.6 and the sample size for second objectives will be 413 which is less than the sample size calculated for second specific objective. Therefore by comparing the sample size for both objectives the final sample size will be 543.where n=the total number of household heads to be interviewed. Therefore, n=543

Table 1: Sample size calculation for second objectives for assessment of street waste management practices and associated factors in Hawassa city, 2019

Objectives	Variable	p-value	Non-response rate (10%)	Total sample size
Dispose solid waste in proper manner in Dire Dawa City	Solid Waste management Practices	31% 31/100=0.31	32	361
Demographic factors in DebreBirhan	family size	OR=0.241 0.24*100=24	28	308
Institutional factors in Bahir Dar	Access to collectors	43% 43/100=0.43	37	413
Socio cultural factors In Addis Ababa	Willingness to pay	78% 78/100=0.78	26	289

3.5.2 Sampling Technique and Procedure

In order to select the study subjects from eight sub city of the Hawassa City. Stratified sampling techniques will be used. First, Eight sub city will be divided in to three strata namely Central (Kebeles close to the center), middle (Kebeles located in the middle distance to the center), and Rural (rural areas of the city).Second, one Kebeles, from each stratum, will be selected using simple random sampling method. In the third stage, households will select proportionally from the three Kebeles based on their population size. Then by using simple RS technique will be used to recruit Household. A representative of 543 households will be selected. For qualitative study, a total of 4 key informants will be purposively selected from the Kebeles solid waste coordinator, staff from Hawassa municipality and Sanitation Beautification Park Development Agency. As shown in (Fig. 3).below:

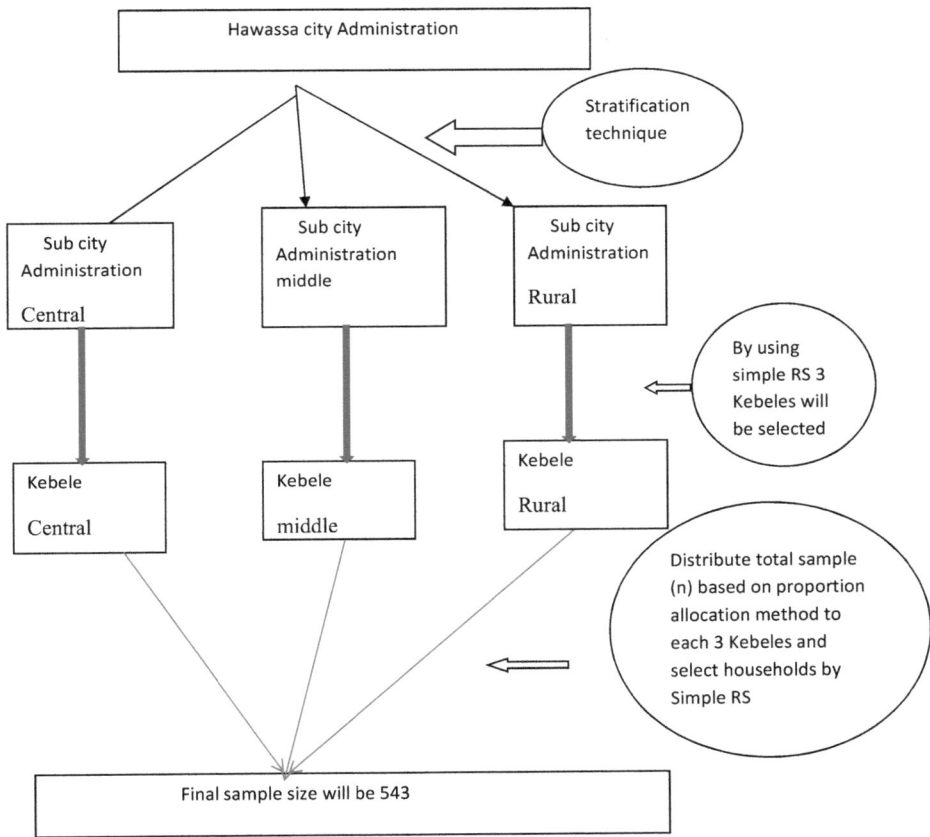

Figure 3: **Schematic representation of sampling procedure of Hawassa city**

3.6. Data collection procedure and quality control

Data will be collected quantitatively using pre-tested and through semi-structured questionnaires administered by way of interviews, Field observations & FGD. The original questionnaires will be prepared by English and translated to local language" Amharic" and latter translate back to English to ensure reliable information. The first draft of the questionnaire will be submitted to the advisor for valuable comments before developing its final version. Questionnaire will be included demographic and socio-economic characteristics, current situation of street solid waste management practices. Interviews will be conducted face to face the data collectors will be trained. Six diploma health workers will be used to collect data and two supervisors will be employed to follow up the data collection process.

3.6.1. Data quality assurance

Pre testing questionnaire will be carried out on HH heads of similar socio demographic characteristics with actual study population, in other than the selected Kebeles considering 5% of total sample size. per to the findings of the pretests, appropriate modifications will be made after discussing with the supervisors and data collectors over their findings of the first hand questions. Two day training will be given for data collectors and supervisors based on the purpose of study and Data collection Procedures. Finally will be checked the questionnaire for completeness and clarity. The principal investigators also will be conduct an active supervision by checking the activities of supervisors and data collectors on randomly bases daily. At least the 5% questionnaires from sample size will be double entered and cleaned for their consistency. The ethical clearance and consent will be secured.

3.7. Variables

3.7. 1.Dependent variables

Street solid waste management practices

3.7.2. Independent variable:

The independent variables will be Demographic factors such as: Sex, Age, Income, Year of stay, Family size and Educational status, Socio-economic factors: Distance from the main road; Willingness to pay for waste collection services; Knowledge about solid waste management, disease transmission; Attitude; Distance from waste containers and Availability of other disposal places and Institutional factor like Man power, Budget, Law of enforcement ,Access to collectors,Availability of container Functionality of vehicle

3.8. Data Analysis

Data will be entered and cleaned using Epi info version 7 and export to SPSS version 21 computer software for further analysis. Frequency and cross tabulations will be used to check for missed value and variable. Descriptive statistics will be carried out to analyze data by using Frequency distribution and percentage of response in each category will be calculated.

Bivariate analysis will be used primarily to check which variable are associated with dependent variable individually.to limit the number of variable and unstable estimates in the subsequent models, only variable p-value less than 0.25 in the Bivariate analysis will further enter into multivariable logistic model. In order to assess the goodness of fit the final model will be checked using Hosmer and Lemeshow. If P value<0.05 will be considered as significant and the Results will be presented in statements, tables, and charts.

3.7. Operational definition:

Household: Persons who live together in one house or dwelling.

Solid waste: all type of solid waste generated from household such as Food related waste,

Municipal solid waste refers to solid waste from houses, streets and public places, shops, offices, and hospitals.

Proper solid waste management at household level: the households store their wastes on covered plastic bag or other material and then hand over to the door to door waste collectors within two to three day.

Door-to-door collections collection of solid waste by micro-enterprises or day laborers who mainly use manually operated carts with "sacks" at least once per week. Ashes, Plastic, Wooden and metallic wastes etc.

Knowledge: the respondent ability to answer the practice of waste management. Hence, those respondents who score 50% and above were considered as having good knowledge toward solid waste management practice. While less than 50% those considered as poor.

Attitude: refer to respondent opinion of agreement or disagreement to the statement concerning waste management. Hence, those respondents who score 50% and above were considered as having good attitude toward solid waste management practice. While those who scored less than 50% were considered as poor.

3.9. Ethical Considerations

Ethical clearance for the proposed research will be obtained from Institutional Review Board (IRB) of Hawassa University College of Medicine and Health Sciences collage school of environmental health. Then a written letter from the university will be obtained and submitted to Hawassa city Municipality. Informed verbal consent will be obtained from each participant before data collection will started. They will also be informed about the confidentiality of the information that is going to be collected. Privacy issue will also assured during the interview for the comfort and confidence of the respondents.

3.10. Disseminating findings

The findings of this study will be presented to Hawassa University School of public and environmental health then it disseminated for all stack holder, Hawassa city Administration municipality, Environmental Protection Agency, Sanitation Beautification and Parks Development Department and it will be also disseminated to other concerned stakeholders.

In addition, all efforts will be used to be publish this paper and appraisal that be written based on the practical exposure.

4. Work plan

Table 2 : shows work plan to accomplish research project in Hawassa town, South Ethiopia, 2019.

Activity	Nov 1	2	3	4	Dec 1	2	3	4	Jan 1	2	3	4	Feb 1	2	3	4	Mar 1	2	3	4	Apr 1	2	3	4	May 1	2	3	4
Preparation of research material																												
development of proposal and submission		▓	▓	▓																								
Proposal defense					▓																							
Submission of revised proposal incorporating the comment of the examiner						▓																						
Submission of ethical request letter							▓																					
Incorporate comments given by ethical committee and getting ethical clearance							▓																					

Select data collectors and supervisors																												
Pre-testing of the survey instrument																												
Data collection																												
Data entry and cleaning																												
Data analysis and interpretation																												
Report writing and submission																												
Thesis defense																												

5. Cost of the Project (Budget)

Table 3: shows the total cost of this master's thesis is estimated to be 30673.10 ETB. Detail cost break down of the project is shown in the table below. Hawassa city, southern, Ethiopia, 2019

S/N	Item description	unit	quantity	Unit price	Number of day	Total price
1	Training					
1.1	Supervisors	Number	2	200	2	800
1.2	Data collector	''	6	300	2	3600
Sub total						4400
2	Stationary and supplies	Number				
2.1	Staples	pack	2	50		100
2.2	Pen	piece	6	10		60
2.3	Pencils	piece	5	10		50
2.4	Eraser	''	5	10		50
2.5	Binder	Pcs	35	10		350
2.6	Paper	Rim	5	250		1250
2.7	Pencil sharpeners	pieces	5	10		50
2.8	Photocopy ,printing and binding					1000
Sub total						2910
3	Field work	unit	quantity	Unit price/day	Number of days	Total price
3.1	Principal investigator	day	1	350	10	3500
3.2	Supervisor	Day	2	300	10	6000
3.3	Data collectors	Day	6	200	10	12000
Sub total						21500
4	Transportation and communication					1500
Sub total	Transportation and communication					1500
Total						30310
Contingency						363.10
Grand total						30673.10

Reference

1.   Zhu D. "Improving Solid Waste Management in India: A Source book for Policy Makers and Practitioners", . The World Bank, Washington DC

(2008).
2.   Amugsi D, Haregu, T, Mberu, B, Muindi, K and Ziraba,. Improving solid waste management practices to reduce health risks in Nairobi and Mombasa June 2018; No. 11. .
3.   Kebede AA, Gezahegn, T., Kololaand, t., & Tsega, W. D. . .Household Solid Waste Generation Rate and Onsite Handling Practices in Debre Berhan Town, Ethiopia. . . Science Journal of Public Health. (2017). ; 5(1)31-34.
4.   TALG(transport accountable local governance) program solid waste management and disposal. Delivery training module 4 The Assia foundation. 2008.
5.   David C. Wilson LR, Modak P, Soos R, Rogero AC, Velis C, Iyer M, et al. United Nations Environment Programme, . 2015.
6.   Ahsan Aa, M and , Shams S. Assessment of Municipal solid waste Management system in Developing countries.chines journal of Engnering Hindawi Publishing Corporation.pp1-11. journal of Engnering Hindawi Publishing Corporation2014.:pp1-11..

7.   USAID (united nation environmental program).Enironmental Guidelines for small scale activities in Africa:(EGSSAA),Solid Waste generation ,handling treatment and disposal. 2009.
8.   Gedefaw M. Assessing the current status of solid waste management of Gondar TownTown, Ethiopia. Int J Sci Technol Res. 2015;4.
9.   "United Nations Economic and Social Commission . Africa Review Report on Waste Management. Committee on Food Security and Sustainable Development Regional Implementation, Addis Ababa, Ethiopia," 2009

10.   hawassa city adminstration munucipal report. 2018.
11.   P. O. U. Adogu, K. A. Uwakwe, N. B. Egenti, A. P. Okwuoha, Nkwocha IB. Assessment of Waste Management Practices among Residents of Owerri Municipal Imo State Nigeria. Journal of Environmental Protection 2015vol. 6,:pp.446-56,.

12.   Yoada RM, Chirawurah D, Adongo PB. Domestic waste disposal practice and perceptions of private sector waste management in urban Accra. BMC Public Health. 2014;14.
13.   Omar AA, Md. Sahadat Hossain, Parvin3 MM. STUDY ON KNOWLEDGE, ATTITUDE AND PRACTICES TOWARDS THE SOLID WASTE MANAGEMENT IN KARAN DISTRICT, MOGADISHU SOMALIA Environmental Contaminants Reviews (ECR) (2018) 1(2): 22-6
14.   Kassahun Ta, Birara E. Assessment of Solid Waste Management Practices in Bahir Dar City, Ethiopia PollutionSpring 2018 4(2)251-61,.

15.   Daniel Shiferaw Alemayehu, Maeregu Seboka Regasa, Bezatu Mengestie, Alemayehu T. Household Solid Waste Management Practice Associated Factors and Service Delivery Performance of Private Solid Waste Collectors in Dire Dawa City, Eastern Ethiopia International Journal of Innovative Research in Science, Engineering and Technology (An ISO 3297: 2007 Certified Organization). October 2017;Vol. 6, Issue 10, (Issue 10,).

16.   Gorfnesh Lema MGM, Amade Eshete and Gizachew Abdeta. Assessment of status of solid waste management in Asella town, Ethiopia BMC Public Health   2019.

17.   Kassa. the Challenges of Solid Waste Management in Urban Areas, the Case of Debremarkos Town. Addis Ababa University, Ethiopia. 2010.
18.   Klunbut P, Aroonsri Mongkolchati, Achara Ussawarujikulchai, Weerawat Ounsaneha, Rattanapan C. Appropriate Option of Market Solid Waste Management based on the Stakeholder Perspectives: A Case Study in a Central Market of Agriculture Products, Thailand Journal of Materials and Environmental Sciences ,2017Volume 8, (Issue 7,): Page 2391-402,.

19.   A w. Determinant of solid waste managment in debrebrhan town American Journal of Theoretical and Applied Statistics. 20019;8,no1:pp 26-30.
20.   . ;Vol. 6, (Issue 10,).

21.   Bamlaku Ayenew AT, Solomon Erifo and Paulos Tesfaye. Household Willingness to Pay for Improved Solid Waste Management in Shashemene Town, Ethiopia. African Journal of Environmental Science and Technology. April 2019 Vol. 13(4), :pp. 162-71, .
22.   SJ Mukui. "Factors influencing household solid waste management in urban Nyeri, Kenya", . Ethiopian Journal of Environmental Studies and Management, . 2013vol.6 no.3, .

23.   Adogu POU, Uwakwe KA, Egenti NB, Okwuoha AP, Nkwocha IB. Assessment of waste management practices among residents of Owerri municipal Imo state Nigeria. J Environ Prot. 2015;6.
24.   BABAYEMI JOD, K. T. . Evaluation of Solid Waste Generation, Categories and Disposal Options in Developing Countries: A Case Study of Nigeria. J Appl Sci Environ Manage September, .Vol. 13(3) 83 - 88

25.   Selamawit Mulat WWaAM. Willingness to pay for improved solid waste management and associated factors among households in Injibara town, Northwest Ethiopia. BMC Res Notes   (2019) (12:401 https://doi.org/10.1186/s13104-019-4433-7).
26.   Shewasinad S, T. D., H. A., N. T. a.& Abera, T. Assessment of Knowledge Attitude and Practice towards Solid and Liquid Waste Management among Addis and Kometa Kebele Community Mizan-Aman Town, Bench – Maji Zone, Snnpr, South Waste Ethiopia, . Science Journal of Public Health (2017). .
27.   klunbut P. Appropriate Option of Market Solid Waste Management based on the Stakeholder Perspectives: A Case Study in a Central Market of Agriculture Products, Thailand Journal of Materials and Environmental Sciences. 2017; Volume 8, (Issue 7,):Page 2391-402.
28.   Getahun T, Beyene M, J AH, Alemayehu E. Municipal solid waste generation in growing urban areas in Africa: Current practices and relation to socioeconomic factors in Jimma, Ethiopia. PubMed. October 2011.
29.   SOLOMON S. Current Solid Waste Management Practices and Problems in Woliata Sodo Town, Southern Ethiopia   J Appl Sci Environ Manage   July 2018 Vol. 22 (7) 1097 –104.

30.   Abiot Abera Aydamo ASNZ, M.I Household solid waste generation rate and physical composition analysis: Case of Hosa'ina city, SNNPRS, Ethiopia J Recent Trends Biosci, . 2012;2(1): 22-28, .
31.   Tadesse.A. Socio Economic Profile of Hyawassa City Administration. . (2013).32.   Cochran's sample size formula,. . 2015.

Hawassa university school of public and Environmental Health

CONSENT OF THE INTERVIEWEE

Hello? I am---------------------from Hawassa University, I am here with my university to study about assess Street Solid Waste Management Practices and associated factories in Hawassa city. We will ask you some questions related to solid waste management practices. Please be assured that the information will be confidential since we do not register names and you may choose to stop your

Participation or refrain from answering any question at any time. If you decide not to participate, your care here will not be affected.

At this time do you ask me anything about this study?

Do I have your agreement to participate----------- (yes or no?)

Signature-------------------

IDENTIFICATION

Interviewer name---------------signature-------------

Supervisor name------------------signature-----------------name of Keble------------

Date of visit-------/-----------/---------Questionnaire number-------------

1. Socio demographic characteristics

Instruction: - in order to answer the following questions, circle your choice.

1. Sex: 1. Male   2. Female

2. Age   1. 18-25 age   2. 26-45 age   3. Over 46

3. Average monthly income: 1. Low income below 500   2. Medium   income between 1000-1500 birr   3. High income above 1500

3. Family size: 1. 1-4 family member   2. 5-8   Family member   3. 9-12 family members

4. Educational level: uneducated   1. No formal education   2. 1-8 Grades complete 3. 9-12 Grades complete above   4. Certificate and above

5. Housing condition   1.private   2.keble   3.rental

6. Occupational status 1.marchent 2.government employer 3.dail labor 4.farmer 5.others

7. Year of stay in Hawassa 1.<1   2.1-5   3.11-15   4.>16

8. Length of stay in current HH (in year) 1.<1   2.1-5   3.5-10   4.>10

9. Distance of HH from main road (in meter) 1.<50   2.500-100   3.101-150   4.>150

10. Availability of space in Back yard for waste disposal 1. yes   2.no

11. Marital status   1/Married   2/ Single   3/ Divorce   4/ Widowed

2. Solid waste management awareness, and practice together with their attitude regarding Solid Waste Management in the city.

1. Are there community solid waste bins in your Keble?   1/yes   2/ no

2. If your answer in 'no' where are dispose or dump solid wastes which are generated from your houses? 1/ everywhere   2/ Land fill   3/ Open space   4/Burning 5/ other

3. If your answer is everywhere what is the reason?   1/ lack of awareness   2/ lack of commitment   3/ lack of SWBs   4/all

4. Do you have SWM and disposal strategies in your house? 1/ yes   2/ no

5. If your answer is yes what are the means of collection and transportation mechanisms? 1/ by using family labor   2/ by using donkey cart or car   3 burning in the compounds   4/ uses other methods

6. Where are you incinerating SWs which is generated from your houses?   1/ in-side the compound   2/ out-side the compound   3/ municipality collect it   4/ dispose in open space, river side and drainage side   5/ uses as energy source

7. The frequency of SW burning practices are   1/ daily   2/ once a week 3/ weekly   4/ I do not know

8. How to manage or handle SWs which are generated from your houses?   1/ collect in closed container   2/ collect open containers   3/ collect by plastic bag 4/ collect by other mechanisms

9. Do you agree improper SW disposal practices affect environment, human life and the ecology? 1/ Yes   2/ No   3/ I do not know

10. Do you agree creating awareness of the community reduce illegal solid waste disposal practices. 1/ agree 2/ strongly agreed   3/ disagree 4/ strongly disagreed

11. Do you know about the rule and regulations with regarding to SWM?

1/ yes   2/no

12. The institutional arrangement of Hawassa city on solid waste management and disposal activity are effective?   1/ Yes   2/ No

13. Do you know the community about the rule and regulation solid waste disposal practices?
1/ yes   2/ no

14. In Hawassa city municipality and sanitation, beautification and parking bureaus implemented integrated solid SWM practices?   1/ yes   2/ no

15. Do you know negative impact of the illegal SW disposal practices? 1/ Yes 2/ No

16. Do you agree the community participate in solid waste management and disposal practices are low?   1/ agree   2/ strongly agree   3/ disagree   4/ strongly disagree

17. Is any private sector, which is, participates on solid waste collection, transportation and dumping activity in Hawassa city?   1/ yes   2/ no

18. Are the following materials like transportation car, waste bins and other equipment's are available in your Keble?   1/ yes   2/ no

19.The town municipality and SBPS are implement the rule and regulation of SWM & proper place disposal by miss behaving individuals and institutions?   1/yes   2/ no

24. is there any alternatives which is reduce improper SW dumping and disposal practices

25. What time do you prefer to dispose your household wastes? (1) Early morning (3) noon (5) early night   (2) Late morning (4) afternoon (6) the time of private waste collectors

26   Do   you   think   solid   wastes   are?(1)   Useless   (3)   useful (2) Somewhat useful

27.Does your household practice waste separation?(1) YES (2) NO

29.If No ,what do you think the reason behind?(1) I do not have the understanding about waste separation(2) I did not think as it is my responsibility(3) I did not visualize the importance of separation(4) if any other reason, please specify it

30. Have you ever come across any form of lesson associated with solid waste management?(1) YES   (2)NO

30.Willingness to pay waste collection services yes/no Access to MSSE service   Enough access   Inadequate   None

31.If your answer for question No. 30 is "YES", through what methods (means) did you get it?(1) In Keble meeting (3) in poster and photograph(2) In health institution (4) if any other

Appendix II

1. Interview Questionnaires Attention: - all the information obtained through this questionnaire shall be uses for the academic purpose only. Anyway, the data collected will be stored, handled and kept confidentially and could not have any effects on the respondents' privacy, and the researcher is fully responsible.

A. Interview for Sanitation, Beautification and parking

1. Poor institutional structure and use inappropriate technologies affected SWM?

2. Is it illegal SWM and disposal practices affect human beings & environment?

3. In Hawassa town how many privet association are organized and participate on SWM and disposed practices?

4. Solid waste storage container or waste bins are found in the town?

5. Briefly discuss about the rule, regulation, its implementation, and monitoring that have been propose by your bureau for efficient practice of SWM in Hawassa town.

6. Discuss about the situation of public awareness and involvement. Existing trends and practices of solid waste management and disposal practices in Hawassa town?

7. What are the main challenges for SWM and disposal practices in Hawassa Town?

B. Interview questionnaires for Municipal managers

1. What are the main causes for poor SWM and disposal Practices?

2. What are the main causes for Poor SWM and disposal Practices in Hawassa town?

3. Is it community and institution participate on SWM and disposal practices?

4. Is it allocates for solid waste management and transportation activity enough budgets and other equipment's?

5. What are the challenges for solid waste management practice in the town?

6. Hawassa town municipality and sanitation sector are enforcing miss behaving individual or institutions?

Appendix III

3. Focus group discussion questionnaires Attention: - all the information obtained through this questionnaire will be uses for the academic purpose only. Always, the data collected will be stored, handled and kept confidentially and could not have any effects on the respondents' privacy and the researcher is fully responsible. To verify this, please do not give your name and any address anywhere in the questionnaire.

A. Sanitation, Beautification and Parking Bureau members

1. How do you see the existing situation of solid waste management & disposal practice?

2. Poor institutional structure and use inappropriate technologies affected SWM?

3. Is it participate community and institutions on SWM and disposal practices?

4. What is the cause for illegal solid waste dumping? In addition, what are the consequences of social, environmental and human impacts of improper solid waste disposal practices?

5. Who is responsible for illegal SWM and disposal practices on everywhere?

6. Are the community knows the rule and regulation of the environmental laws?

7. in the town how many privet associations found in your town?

8. Solid waste storage container or waste bins are found in the town?

B. Purposively selected Kebele leaders & Households (FGD)

1. Solid waste disposal site selection is appropriate for disposal activities? Elaborate?

2. Community involvement in SWM and disposal practices is effective or not?

3. is the town municipality and sanitation, beautification create awareness about solid SWM and disposal practices? Elaborate

4. Do you know the rule and regulation of SWM and environmental law?

5. How to handle solid waste that generate from your houses. Is it the best way?

6. What is the challenge for SWM and disposal practices in your locality?

7. Do you know the impact of illegal solid waste management and disposal practices?

Interviewer name-------   supervisor name-------------

Signature-----------   signature--------------

Please thank the interviewee for his/her participation-------------

Appendix IV Structured Observation

The practices of solid waste management and disposal practices in Hawassa city

1. Presence of solid waste containers

2. Current practices of solid waste management and disposal practices

3. Current trends of solid waste management and disposal practices

4. Solid waste disposal site and transportation equipment

5. Other visual practices in the town.

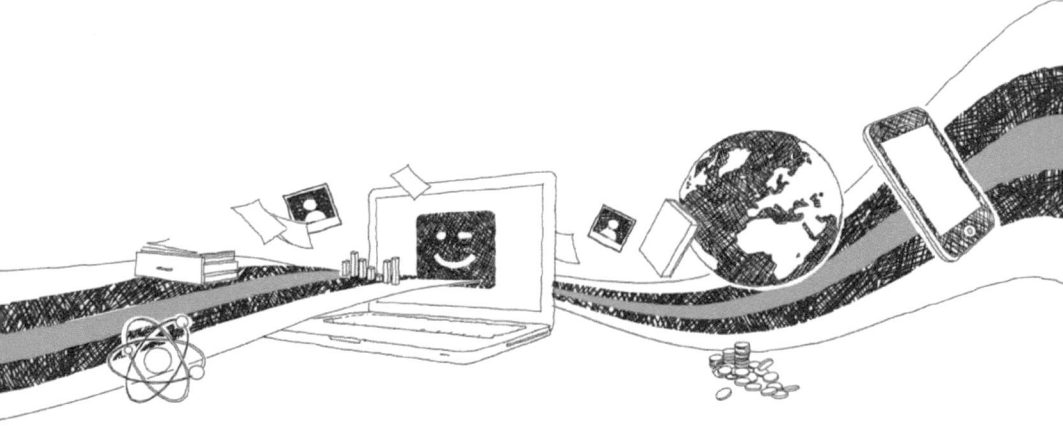
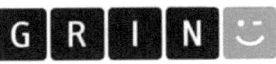